# Culturally Sensitive Care of Individuals with Intellectual and Developmental Disabilities

Anne Hedelius, M.A., L.S.W., B.A.S.W.

- Define language and terminology
- Discuss the shift from institutionalized care to community-based services.
- Gain competencies in the barriers that contribute to inequities in health care.
- Recommended interventions

- The importance of family support

- The term mental retardation has fallen out of favor due to its history of derogatory use and the preference of individuals with disabilities for specific language to describe their limitations.
- The preferred terminology is intellectual disabilities (ID), developmental disabilities (DD), or cognitive impairments (Parish & Saville, 2006).

- Individuals with ID have a vulnerability that places them at risk for unfavorable health and well-being outcomes (Parish & Ellison-Martin, 2007; Wallace & Beange, 2008).
- Individuals with ID often have co-morbidities that require more frequent use of health care (Jansen, Krol, Groothoff, & Post, 2004; Liptak, Stuart, & Auinger, 2006).

- DD is defined in the Developmental Disabilities Assistance and Bill of Rights Act of 2000, as substantial

- functional limitations in three or more domains (HHS).
- The term DD applies to individuals with chronic deficits in social, emotional, intellectual, and physical development appearing before the age of 22 (McCallion & Nickle, 2008; Parish & Lutwick, 2005).

Many individuals with ID and DD suffer additional disabilities, restricting their mobility, communication, and access to health care (Betz, Baer, Poulsen, Vahanvaty, & Bare, 2004).

- Individuals with disabilities share a history of devaluation, limitations of civil rights, marginalization, and oppression.
- "Disabled individuals confront race, class, and gender discrimination as well" (Gilson & Depoy, 2000)
- Shared language, social networks, and systems of support, counter negative influences from society.

- In the early seventies, community advocates, families, national organizations, and political activists exposed abuses and demanded community-based care (Mansell, 2006; Parish, 2005).
- Deinstitutionalization and normalization of disabilities within the community led to a shift in attitudes, viewing social and environmental barriers as the problem instead of the individual with a disability (Fujiura & Parish, 2007; Jansen et al., 2004).

- Changes in federal laws required states to develop community based services that supported an individual's ability to live in their own home (Mansell, 2006; Parish, 2005).
- The majority of individuals with ID and DD can live at home with appropriate support.
- Preventative health care services can be provided in the home or community at a lower cost (Betz et al., 2004; Hiebert-Murphy, Trute, & Wright, 2008; McGinty, Worthington & Dennison, 2008; Mansell, 2006; Parish, Rose, Andrews, & Shattuck, 2009; Porterfield & McBride, 2007; Wallace & Beange, 2008).

- Early intervention programs provide in-home therapeutic

services for age zero to three (Individuals with Disabilities Education Act part C, 2004; McGinty et al., 2008)

- Therapeutic services are provided in public schools for ages three to twenty-one (Individuals with Disabilities Education Act, part B, 2004)
- Medicaid waivers, often known as Katie Beckett waivers, are available in every state to support in-home care of children who might otherwise require nursing home placement (Parish et al., 2009).

- Improvements in medical technology and the influence of managed care shifted the burden of care out of institutions and into the community (Jansen et al., 2004; Parish, Moss, & Richman, 2008)

## Nationally

Two in every seven families in the United States, have a family member with a disability. In 2000, 49.7 million people reported having a long lasting disability, and among these, 12.4 million reported cognitive limitations (U.S. Census).

**2 in 7 families are affected**

- In 2000, more than ten million people reported a need for in-home services to accomplish activities of daily living (U.S. Census).

- In the year 2000, the United States allocated $29 billion for all types of developmental disabilities spending, of that amount only one billion was spent for in-home family support services; the vast majority of spending was on institutionalized care (Parish & Lutwick, 2005).

- More than 60% of individuals with intellectual and developmental disabilities live at home with their families (Parish & Lutwick, 2005).
- As people age, the risk of disability increases and experts

contend that the over age 65 population will more than double by 2050 (U.S. Census, 2000).

- Individuals with intellectual and developmental disabilities are at high risk of institutionalization.
- Institutionalization results in increased costs and displacement from families and the community.
- Community-based services must consistently demonstrate superior outcomes when compared to institutionalized services (Mansell, 2006).

Providing effective supports maintains family integrity and prevents costly out-of-home placements in order to obtain needed care (Jansen, et al., 2004).

- A commitment to helping individuals and their families with obtaining equitable services, that are individualized, client directed, culturally relevant, and that promote optimal health & wellness (AAIDD, 2002; CMSA, 2002; IOM, 2007; WHO, 2008).
- Federal laws mandate the equitable treatment of individuals with cognitive

disabilities. The civil rights of individuals with disabilities are protected by Section 504 of the Rehabilitation Act of 1973 (U.S. Dept. of Justice, 2005)

- Epilepsy
- Obesity
- Cardiovascular disease
- Osteoporosis
- Hypothyroidism
- Diabetes
- Mobility issues
- Visual impairments
- Sensory impairments
- Dental decay


- Early-onset senile dementia

- Gastroesophageal disease
- Breast and cervical cancers
- Respiratory disease
- Language disorders
- Psychiatric and behavioral disorders
- Hearing loss

- Inadequate implementation of the Americans with Disabilities Act (IOM, 2007)
- Limitations of insurance plans, Medicaid & Medicare (Burns, 2009; IOM, 2007; Parish & Ellison-Martin, 2007)
- Gaps in insurance coverage occur when individuals reach adulthood and transition to adult services (IOM, 2007)
- Research remains underfunded and public policy has been slow to change (IOM, 2007; Parish et al., 2008)

- The U.S. liberal market-based economy seeks to cut health care costs
- Current trends propose rationing of services, de-differentiation of those with disabilities, and the elimination of special categories of care (Mansell, 2006).
- Need for cost savings to secure the support of policy makers should not oversimplify the needs of those with ID & DD (Mansell, 2006).

- Health care reform seeks to cut health care costs

- Decisions driven by tax payers rather than by consumers of services
- Managed care
- Provide minimal care at lowest cost
- Access to services only in crisis
- Reduces cost-sharing between individuals with disabilities and the community

- Replaces specialist models with generic models
- Eliminates specialized categories of care
- General services may overlook individual needs
- Greater competition for resources

- " De-differentiation is the loss of special, separate policies and service structures for people with intellectual disabilities and their replacement with general policies and structures" (Mansell, 2006, p. 72).

- Rights-based model of disability services
- Oversimplification, assumption that the disabled community can represent itself
- Fails to acknowledge the inability of individuals with ID & DD to effectively advocate for themselves
- "the rise of the social model has also served to de-emphasize the

impairments people with disabilities have" (Mansell, 2006, p. 72).

- Views disability as a permanent biological impediment
- The problem is within the individual
- In need of rehabilitation or adaptation
- Biological determinism: focus is on "physical, behavioral, psychological, cognitive, and sensory tragedy" (Gilson & Depoy, 2000).

- Care tends to take longer and needs are more complex
- Majority of health care providers lack specialized training in ID & DD (McGinty et al., 2008; Melville et al., 2005; Mott, Chau, & Chan, 2007; Wallace & Beange, 2008)
- Some providers have stereotypical bias towards those with disabilities (Burns, 2009; Parish & Saville, 2006; Wallace & Beange, 2008)
- Amplified risk of not having medical needs recognized resulting in death and neglect (Wallace & Beange, 2008)

- In 2007, The American College of Obstetricians and Gynecologists recommended that prenatal testing for cognitive disabilities be made available to

all pregnant women (ACOG, 2007 as cited in Bauer, 2008).
- Attempts to avoid human suffering may exacerbate the devaluation of individuals with cognitive disabilities (Bauer, 2008).
- If cognitive disabilities are perceived as preventable, society may become reluctant to fund needed services.


- Stereotypes and prejudices are based on a history of institutionalization.
- Older individuals with ID and DD never had the benefit of current medical

technology and community-based services.
- A need exists for up-to-date and unbiased information about the potential of individuals with cognitive disabilities (Bauer, 2008).

- Women have been the traditional caregivers of individuals with ID and DD.

- Changing demographics of American families have reduced the availability of women as caregivers (Fujiura and Parish, 2007; McCallion & Nickle, 2008)
- Shifts burden of care to the community
- Service needs for custodial care are in direct competition with systems serving other elderly populations (Fujiura and Parish, 2007).

- Shortage of qualified workers in the community
- Leads to problems with continuity of care
- Attention to medical history and need for preventative

care is often overlooked (Parish & Ellison-Martin, 2007; Parish & Saville, 2006; McGinty et al., 2008).

- Need exists for professionals to specialize in cognitive disabilities in all areas of health care and human services (Wallace & Beange, 2008).

- High correlation of poverty, social problems, mental disturbance, and chronic illnesses associated with ID and DD (Jansen et al., 2004; Liptak et al., 2006; McCallion & Nickle, 2008; Parish & Lutwick, 2005; Parish et al., 2009; Porterfield & McBride, 2007; Wallace and Beange, 2008).

- Existing community supports are inadequate to meet the growing needs of the disabled population (Fujiura & Parish, 2007; Parish & Lutwick 2005; McCallion & Nickle 2008; Wallace & Beange, 2008).
- Caregivers experience more stress and are at increased risk for developing depression and health care concerns (Betz et al., 2004; McGinty et al., 2008).

- Families report difficulty in accessing specialty medical and therapeutic services (McGinty et al., 2008; Porterfield & McBride, 2007).
- Children with ID and DD experience more frequent illnesses and absenteeism

- from school (Betz et al., 2004; Liptak et al., 2006).
- Despite the advances of federal laws, individuals and their families continue to face discrimination and prejudice (Castaneto & Willemsen, 2006).

- Person centered care planning requires the participation of the client with ID and the incorporation of their individual needs (Wallace & Beange, 2008).
- Much of what is known about individuals with ID is based on caregiver statements and observation, rather than on self reports (Parish et al., 2008).

- How to identify barriers and personalize interventions when it is not possible to solicit the collective desires of individuals.

The question faced by health care workers is how to best deliver services based on current policy and budget constraints in a way that achieves optimal health and wellness outcomes for clients.

# Strategies for Change for Advanced Practice Nurses

- Critical changes can and must be made (Wallace & Beange, 2008)
- Professional attitudes are pivotal towards creating change (Castaneto & Willemsen, 2006; IOM, 2007; Mansell, 2006)
- Position statements state the standard of care (AAIDD, 2002; CMSA, 2002; IOM, 2007; WHO, 2008)
- The changes made in the past four decades came about in part through the advocacy of health care and human services (Mansell, 2006; Parish, 2005)

- Bring client needs to the attention of stakeholders in the health care arena.
- Demonstrate a cost savings in order to secure the support of policymakers (Burns, 2009; Fujiura & Parish, 2007; Mansell, 2006)
- Initiate change at agency, state, and federal levels (Fujiura & Parish, 2007; Parish et al., 2009)
- Represent client needs in political and professional forums (McGinty et al., 2008)

- Empower families to care for their family members with disabilities (McGinty et al., 2008)

- Through coordination of services, timely acquisition of services, and supporting the families stated goals (Hiebert-Murphy et al., 2008)
- Clarify agency roles and functions, helping families to become discerning consumers.
- Provide emotional support in addition to concrete services (McGinty et al., 2008)

- Education and awareness of available services should commence with the diagnosis of a disability.
- Encourage self-advocacy skills by connecting families to support groups, internet

websites, and reading materials (McGinty et al., 2008).
- Assist in understanding the often conflicting goals and agendas of multiple agencies (McGinty et al., 2008).

- Develop partnerships with families, promoting decision making, mastery of care, and fostering self-determination (CMSA, 2002; McGinty et al., 2008; NASW n.d.)
- Family centered practice requires the use of a strengths model
- Take the time to focus on successes (McGinty et al., 2008)

- Health care workers should be well educated in the grieving and adjustment that accompanies the diagnosis of a cognitive disability and the fact that this is an evolving process.
- Families often suffer repeated losses throughout the years as they come to terms with the limitations of the disability (Hiebert-Murphy et al., 2008; McCallion & Nickle, 2008; McGinty et al., 2008).

- Help families with long term planning, guardianship, and

information about future challenges.
- Advanced practice nurses (APN) must gain competencies in tackling the difficult issues of guardianship and advance directives (McCallion & Nickle, 2008)

- Be familiar with all systems of care including health care, mental health, developmental disabilities, vocational rehabilitation, insurance plans, state, and community agencies (McGinty et al., 2008).

- Link families to specialists and assist with the transition to adult services (McGinty et al., 2008; Porterfield & McBride, 2007).

- Specialized education on the needs of the disabled population should be offered at all points of entry for workers in the human services and health care fields (IOM, 2007; Melville et al., 2005).
- The IOM further recommends that, "federal agencies should launch a major public information campaign to increase professional and consumer awareness" (2007, p. 3).

Educational programs should be implemented in medical and nursing schools to prepare new graduates to meet the needs of the population with ID & DD (Tracy & Iacono, 2008; Wallace & Beange, 2006).

Health care professionals need focused training on communication techniques and the unique health care needs of the population with disabilities (Melville et al., 2005).

- APN can offer formal and informal supports that will improve the quality of care.

- Establish protocols for referrals and follow-up (Hiebert-Murphy et al., 2008; Wallace & Beange, 2008).
- Education
- Active support of the health care team.

- Facilitate and review care plans and discharges
- Provide consultation to general practitioners, and establish standards of care
- Establish guidelines for risk management and quality control (Wallace & Beange, 2008)

- Active support is associated with improved staff performance and improved health care outcomes (Mansell, 2006; Melville et al., 2005).
- Advocate for patients by ruling out medical reasons for behaviors and planning interventions to manage disruptive behaviors (Hiebert-Murphy et al., 2008; McGinty et al., 2008).

- Health care access for individuals with ID & DD can be improved through effective case management techniques, specialization,

education, and political activism.
- APN can meet the need for specialization by staying current with the research, understanding the systems of care, and advocating for program expansion.

Through advocacy, APN can encourage families and individuals to become politically active, representing their needs at the community, state, and federal level.

Exciting opportunities exist for creative individuals to develop educational materials, policies, and programs to meet needs within the health care industry for innovative approaches to improving quality of care for the disabled population.

AAIDD. (2009). *Service coordination*. Retrieved February 15, 2010, from http://www.aamr.org/content_167.cfm?navID=31

Bauer, P. E. (2008). "Tell them it's not so bad": Prenatal screening for Down syndrome and the bias toward abortion. *Intellectual and Developmental Disabilities, 46*(3), 247-251. doi:10.1352/2008.46:247-251

Betz, C. L., Baer, M. T., Poulsen, M., Vahanvaty, U., & Bare, M. (2004). Secondary analysis of primary and preventative services accessed and perceived service barriers by children with developmental disabilities and their families. *Issues in Comprehensive Pediatric Nursing, 27*, 83-106. doi:10.1080/01460860490451813

Burns, M. E. (2009). Medicaid managed care and health care access for adult beneficiaries with disabilities. *Health Services Research, 44 (5p1),* 1521-1541. doi:10.1111/j.1475-6773.2009.00991.x

Case Management Society of America. (2002). *CMSA's standards of practice for case management.* Retrieved February 15, 2010, from http://www.cmsa.org/Individual/MemberToolkit/StandardsofPractice/tabid/69/Default.aspx

Castaneto, M. V., & Willemsen, E. W. (2006). Social perception of the development of disabled children. *Child: Care, Health and Development, 33*(3), 308-318. doi:10.1111/j.1365-2214.2006.00675.x

Fujiura, G. T., & Parish, S. L. (2007). Emerging policy challenges in intellectual disabilities. *Mental Retardation and Developmental Disabilities, 13,* 188-194. doi:10.1002/mrdd.20152

Gilson, S.F., & Depoy, E. (2000), Multiculturalism and disability: a critical perspective. *Disability & Society,* 15(2), 207-218.

Hiebert-Murphy, D., Trute, B., & Wright, A. (2008). Patterns of entry to community-based services for families with children with developmental disabilities: Implications for social work practice. *Child and Family Social Work, 13,* 423-432. doi:10.1111/j.1365-2206.2008.00572.x

Individuals with Disabilities Education Act. (2004). Retrieved March 9, 2010, from http://idea.ed.gov/

Institute of Medicine. (2007). *The future of disability in America.* Retrieved February 16, 2010, from http://www.iom.edu/Reports/2007/The-Future-of-Disability-in-America.aspx

Jansen, D. E., Krol, B., Groothoff, J. W., & Post, D. (2004). People with intellectual disability and their health problems: A review of comparative studies. *Journal of Intellectual Disability Research, 48*(2), 93-102.

Liptak, G. S., Stuart, T., & Auinger, P. (2006). Health care utilization and expenditures for children with autism: Data from U.S. national samples. *Journal of Autism & Developmental Disorders, 36,* 871-879. doi:10.1007/s40803-006-0119-9

Mansell, J. (2006). Deinstitutionalization and community living: Progress, problems and priorities. *Journal of Intellectual & Developmental Disability, 31*(2), 65-76. doi:10.1080/j.36682500600686726

McCallion, P., & Nickle, T. (2008). Individuals with developmental disabilities and their caregivers. In S. M. Cummings & N.P. Kropf (Eds.), *Handbook of Psychosocial Interventions with Older Adults: Evidence-Based Approaches* (pp. 245-266). doi:10.1080/01634370802137959

McGinty, K., Worthington, R., & Dennison, W. (2008). Patient and family advocacy: Working with individuals with comorbid mental illness and developmental disabilities and their families. *Psychiatric Quarterly, 79,* 193-203. doi:10.1007/s44426-008-9075-4

Melville, C. A., Cooper, S. A., Morrison, J., Finlayson, J., Allan, L., Robinson, N., Martin, G. (2005). The outcomes of an intervention study to reduce the barriers experienced by people with intellectual disabilities accessing primary health care services. *Journal of Intellectual Disability Research, 50*(1), 11-17. doi:10.1111/j.1365-2788.2005.00719.x

Mott, S., Chau, A., & Chan, J. (2007). Meeting the health needs of people with disability living in the community. *Journal of Intellectual & Developmental Disability, 32*(1), 51-53. doi:10.1080/j.3668250601184697

Parish, S. L. (2005). Deinstitutionalization in two states: the impact of advocacy, policy, and other social forces on services for people with developmental disabilities. *Research & Practice for Persons with Severe Disabilities, 30*(4), 219-231.

Parish, S. L., & Ellison-Martin, M. J. (2007). Health-care access of women Medicaid recipients. *Journal of Disability Policy Studies, 18*(2), 109-116.

Parish, S. L., & Lutwick, Z. E. (2005). A critical analysis of the emerging crisis in long-term care for people with developmental disabilities. *Social Work, 50*(4), 345-354.

Parish, S. L., Moss, K., & Richman, E. L. (2008). Perspectives on health care of adults with developmental disabilities. *Intellectual and Developmental Disabilities, 46*(6), 411-426. doi:10.1352/2008.46 :411-426

Parish, S. L., Rose, R. A., Andrews, M. E., & Shattuck, P. T. (2009). Receipt of professional care coordination among families raising children with special health care needs: A multilevel analysis of state policy needs. *Children and Youth Services Review, 31,* 63-70. doi:10.1016/j.childyouth.2008.05.010

Parish, S. L., & Saville, A. W. (2006). Women with cognitive limitations living in the community: Evidence of disability-based disparities in health care. *Mental Retardation, 44*(4), 249-259.

Porterfield, S. L., & McBride, T. D. (2007). The effect of poverty and caregiver education on perceived need and access to health services among children with special health care needs. *American Journal of Public Health, 97*(2), 323-329.

Tracy, J., & Iacono, T. (2008). People with developmental disabilities teaching medical students: Does it make a difference? *Journal of Intellectual & Developmental Disability, 33*(4), 345-348. doi:10.1080/j.3668250802478633

U.S. Census Bureau. (2000). *United States Census 2000.* Retrieved January 27, 2010, from http://www.census.gov/main/www/cen2000.html

U.S. Department of Health & Human Services. (2000). *Administration for children & families.* Retrieved February 15, 2010, from http://www.acf.hhs.gov/programs/add/ddact/DDACT2.html

U.S. Department Of Justice. (2005, September). *A Guide to Disability Rights Law.* Retrieved May 17, 2010, from http://www.ada.gov/cguide.htm

Wallace, R. A., & Beange, H. (2008). On the need for a specialist service within the geriatric hospital setting for the adult patient with intellectual disability and physical health problems. *Journal of Intellectual & Developmental Disability, 33*(4), 354-361. doi:10.1080/j.3668250802259264

World Health Organization. (2008). *Entry into force of the Convention on the Rights of Persons with Disabilities.* Retrieved February 16, 2010, from http://www.who.int/nmh/media/speeches/adg_statement_april_2008/en/index.html

Made in the USA
Columbia, SC
10 May 2023